HERBAL REMEDIES FOR COUGH

Breathe Easy With Herbal Solutions To Explore Targeted Healing, Targeting Respiratory Relief, Key Focus Areas, And The Magic Of Nature's Remedies

DR. CARDEN KYRIE

DISCLAIMER

The only goal of this book is informational. Every effort has been taken by the author and publisher to ensure that the information provided is accurate. But the material in this book is given "as is," without any express or implied representation, warranty, or condition as to its accuracy, completeness, or suitability for any particular purpose.

Any loss, damage, or injury resulting from using the information in this book, or from any action or decision made as a result of such use, will not be covered by the author's or publisher's liability. It is recommended that readers seek the assistance of a certified specialist for guidance specific to their situation.

The opinions and viewpoints conveyed in this book belong to the author and may not necessarily represent the official stance or policies of any specified organizations or people. Any likeness to real-life occurrences, places, or people—living or deceased—is wholly coincidental.

No specific product, service, or therapy discussed in this book is endorsed by the author or publisher. Any reference to goods or services is made only for informative reasons and is not intended as a recommendation or endorsement.

Before making any judgments or acting on any information, readers are urged to independently confirm it all. Any unfavorable effects or repercussions arising from the usage of the material included in this book are disclaimed by the author and publisher.

By using this book, you consent to absolving the publisher and author of any and all claims, obligations, or losses resulting from your use of the material in it.

I appreciate your cooperation and understanding.

TABLE OF CONTENTS

CHAPTER ONE
INTRODUCTION TO HERBAL COUGH MEDICINES

RECOGNIZING COUGHS

Coughs are a common respiratory ailment that can be brought on by several things, including environmental irritants and infections. Investigating and using successful herbal medicines requires an understanding of the nature of coughs. The body's natural response to remove foreign objects, mucus, or irritants from the airways is a cough. It is usually characterized by a strong coughing motion that is frequently accompanied by a characteristic noise.

COUGH TYPES

Coughs come in various varieties, each with unique traits and underlying reasons. A dry cough can be brought on by irritation or inflammation in the throat and is typically non-productive, meaning it doesn't create mucus. A productive or wet cough, on the other hand, involves the discharge of mucus and is frequently linked to respiratory illnesses like the flu or the common cold. Furthermore, persistent coughs that continue longer than eight weeks may be a sign of underlying medical issues such as allergies, asthma, or gastro esophageal reflux disease (GERD).

REASONS FOR COUGHING

Many different things might irritate or inflame the respiratory system, which can lead to coughing. Acute coughs are mostly caused by respiratory illnesses, such as bacterial or viral diseases. Allergens and environmental irritants such as smoke, dust, or pollutants can also cause coughing.

Chronic coughs can be caused by long-term illnesses like bronchitis, asthma, or even side effects from medications. Customizing a suitable treatment for a cough requires knowing its exact etiology.

Herbal cough treatments are becoming more and more well-liked as a safer, more natural substitute for prescription cough drops. Many herbs have qualities that help calm the respiratory tract, reduce inflammation, and support good respiratory health in general. Herbs that are frequently used to treat coughs include thyme, which has antibacterial qualities, and licorice root, which has anti-inflammatory and expectorant qualities. Because they are calming and antibacterial, peppermint, ginger, and honey are also commonly used.

THE VALUE OF EFFICIENT COUGH RELIEF

Beyond just making you feel better, good cough treatment is crucial since chronic coughing can cause other issues like weariness, insomnia, and strained chest muscles. Furthermore, a persistent cough can make daily tasks more difficult and negatively affect a person's general quality of life. Herbal treatments help the body's natural healing processes in addition to treating the symptoms, improving respiratory health, and averting more difficulties.

Investigating the world of herbal cough cures requires an awareness of the nature of coughs, the types and reasons for them, and the importance of effective relief. Through the use of the medicinal qualities of different herbs, people can look for natural remedies that help with respiratory system health overall as well as symptom relief.

CHAPTER TWO

OVERVIEW OF HERBAL MEDICINE

HERBAL MEDICINE'S PAST

Phytotherapy, plant medicine, and herbal medicine have a long and varied history spanning many centuries and civilizations. The development of human cultures and their pursuit of health and well-being are closely linked to the history of herbal medicine. Herbal therapy has its origins in ancient civilizations when local people learned about the therapeutic qualities of plants by trial and error. History demonstrates that several civilizations, such as China, India, Egypt, and Greece, created advanced herbal medicine systems.

Herbal medicine had a significant role in traditional Chinese medicine (TCM) in ancient China when practitioners placed a strong emphasis on the harmony of Qi, Yin, and Yang, the body's vital forces. Herbal treatment was also accepted by traditional Indian medicine, or Ayurveda, which focused on balancing body functions and individual constitutions. On papyrus scrolls, the Egyptians documented their knowledge of medicinal plants, while Greek physicians such as Hippocrates documented the application of herbs in medicine.

FUNDAMENTALS OF HERBAL MEDICINE

The holistic approach to health and wellness is fundamental to the ideas of herbal treatment. Herbalists see health as a condition of balance because they recognize the connection between the body, mind, and spirit. The idea of employing the entire plant for medical reasons is one of the guiding principles. Herbal therapy depends on the synergy of different plant constituents, in contrast to current medications that frequently isolate and synthesize specific molecules, with the belief that the combined action improves therapeutic effects.

Additionally, herbalists stress the value of customized care. Since every person is different, herbal medicines are frequently customized to meet each person's particular needs and constitution. This tailored approach contrasts sharply with the one-size-fits-all paradigm commonly linked to traditional medicine. Another important component is the idea of preventative medicine, which supports the use of herbs to preserve general health and stave off disease.

SAFETY POINTS TO REMEMBER

Safety concerns must come first, even with herbal medicine's advantages and track record of success. Despite being natural materials, herbs do carry some hazards. Both herbalists and consumers need to be aware of possible risks such as toxicity, allergic responses, and interactions with prescription medications. Purchasing herbs from reliable vendors is essential to guarantee their quality and purity. Herbal safety also heavily depends on dosage and administration, since incorrect use can have unfavorable effects.

In addition, the absence of uniform regulations in the herbal medicine sector highlights how crucial it is to consult with licensed professionals. Herbalists are knowledgeable enough to handle the complexity of herbal medicines, guaranteeing both safety and efficacy because they frequently receive substantial training. To prevent possible conflicts with conventional medical procedures, users are advised to be transparent in their communication with healthcare experts regarding any herbal medicines they may be taking.

The history of herbal medicine is a tapestry woven with the strands of cultural traditions and old wisdom. Herbal medicine is based on a holistic view of health, with a focus on using whole herbs and creating customized remedies. The necessity for careful and educated use, directed by the knowledge of certified professionals, is highlighted by the safety concerns surrounding herbal medicine.

CHAPTER THREE

HOW TO CHOOSE AND USE HERBS
RECOGNIZING USEFUL HERBS

Herbal identification is a technique that combines intuition, observation, and knowledge. To effectively identify herbs, one needs to be familiar with their distinct qualities, including look, fragrance, and taste. Herbalist books, field guides, and internet resources can all be very helpful in this attempt since they offer comprehensive information and illustrations to help identify different plants.

It's also essential to comprehend the unique characteristics and applications of plants. Beneficial herbs can be used for a variety of tasks, including medical and culinary ones. Herbs such as basil, rosemary, and thyme, for example, are used in cooking and have therapeutic qualities. Gaining a thorough grasp of the health benefits associated with each herb empowers people to make well-informed decisions about integrating them into their everyday routines.

DEVELOPING AND GATHERING HERBS

Herb cultivation is a fulfilling undertaking that calls for close attention to soil quality, environmental factors, and adequate maintenance. Many herbs grow best in well-drained soil with lots of sunshine, and good herb cultivation requires knowing what each particular herb needs. Whether growing herbs in pots, on a windowsill, or in a garden, the appropriate growing conditions encourage optimum growth and guarantee a plentiful crop.

Timely harvesting of herbs is essential for maintaining their flavor and therapeutic qualities. Herbs are usually best collected right before they flower because that's when their essential oils are at their highest concentration. To prevent harming the plant, harvesting should be done using sharp scissors or pruning shears.

Additionally, regular pruning promotes bushier growth, which increases the yield of the plant.

APPROPRIATE PREPARATION AND STORAGE

Herb potency preservation involves not only growing them in the garden but also using the right storage and preparation methods. Herbs can be preserved in their flavor and medicinal properties by drying them. Herbs can be effectively dried by air drying, using a dehydrator, or hanging bundles in a cool, dark spot. To preserve their freshness, herbs should be kept out of direct sunlight and heat in sealed containers.

To prepare herbs correctly, one must be aware of the intended culinary or medicinal use. Herbs can be chopped, minced, or infused into oils or vinegar for culinary purposes to improve the flavor of food. Making teas, tinctures, or salves with meticulous attention to dosage and preparation techniques may be necessary for medicinal uses.

The process of choosing and utilizing herbs is a comprehensive one that includes harvesting, identification, cultivation, and safe handling. Through the development of these skills and knowledge, people can fully utilize the therapeutic and culinary potential of beneficial plants.

CHAPTER FOUR

COMMON HERBS TO ALLEVIATE COUGH

CALM HERBS

Calming herbs are a safe, all-natural way to ease respiratory discomfort and have long been known for their ability to relieve coughs. Licorice root is one of the most effective of these. The Glycyrrhiza glabra plant yields licorice root, which has anti-inflammatory and sedative qualities due to its constituents. These ingredients aid in relieving inflamed respiratory tract and throat mucous membranes. Furthermore, licorice root has been linked to encouraging the formation of good mucus, which may help relieve dry, bothersome coughs.

MARSHMALLOW ROOT

Marshmallow root is another plant well known for its calming properties on coughs. Marshmallow root, which is extracted from the Althaea officinalis plant, includes mucilage, a gel-like material that coats injured tissues to provide protection. This coating effect soothes cough reflexes and lessens discomfort in the throat. Marshmallow root's expectorant qualities are partly attributed to its mucilaginous texture, which aids in the removal of mucus from the respiratory system.

SLIPPERY ELM

Another helpful herb for treating coughs is slippery elm. For centuries, people have utilized the inner bark of the Ulmus rubra tree, also called slippery elm, for its calming properties. Similar to marshmallow and licorice roots, slippery elm soothes inflamed tissues by creating a protective layer that eases coughing and sore throats. It is also thought to promote mucus production, which helps to protect and repair the respiratory system.

The potential of these three herbs—licorice root, marshmallow root, and slippery elm—to calm and shield the respiratory system is something they all have in common.

They are useful partners in the treatment of both dry and wet coughs due to their calming qualities. As herbal treatments, they provide a mild method of relieving coughs without the unpleasant side effects that are sometimes connected to synthetic cough medications.

ROOT LICORICE

Particularly licorice root has been studied for its antiviral qualities, making it a useful herb for cough reduction as well as respiratory health support in general. However, it is imperative to consume licorice root with caution because overindulging in it might have negative effects including raised blood pressure.

On the other hand, slippery elm and marshmallow root are generally well tolerated and safe to use. Their long history of use in many cultures attests to their efficacy and safety in relieving coughs and sore throats. Adding these calming herbs to herbal teas, infusions, or preparations can provide a comprehensive and all-natural way to treat cough symptoms.

Three prominent examples of calming herbs are slippery elm, marshmallow root, and licorice root; each offers special qualities to ease coughs and calm irritated respiratory tracts. Their potential as useful instruments in the quest for natural cough alleviation is highlighted by their lengthy history of usage in traditional medicine and the expanding corpus of research on their advantages.

ANTI-IMMUNE HERBS

Improving the immune system is essential for fighting coughs, and several herbs are known to strengthen the immune system. Among the herbs that have been traditionally used to strengthen the immune system is echinacea. Its active ingredients are thought to increase immune cell synthesis, enhancing the body's defenses against infections. Another herb with immune-modulating properties is astragalus. It is believed to strengthen the body's defenses against different infections, which may lessen the intensity and length of coughs.

The well-known immune-stimulating plant elderberry has a long history of use in traditional medicine. Elderberry, which is high in antioxidants, is thought to support immune protection by preventing viruses from reproducing within the body. By strengthening the body's natural defenses, the combination of these immune-boosting herbs may offer a comprehensive method of supporting the body during coughs.

ANTIBACTERIAL PLANTS

Using antimicrobial herbs not only strengthens the immune system but also directly fights the germs that cause coughing. Thyme is a fragrant plant that's often used in cooking. Its essential oils, such as thymol, are said to have antibacterial qualities. Thyme has been used to treat respiratory conditions and, by attacking germs and viruses, may also aid with cough symptoms.

Another culinary herb that has antibacterial properties is oregano, which is abundant in substances like carvacrol. It has been used historically for respiratory ailments and, by addressing the underlying microbiological causes of coughs, may help relieve them. Allicin, a substance with strong antibacterial qualities, is found in garlic, which is recognized for its strong flavor and scent. Garlic is a great herb for cough alleviation because it has been used for ages to treat a variety of health issues, including respiratory infections.

People may benefit from these antimicrobial herbs' capacity to target the bacteria that cause coughs, offering both symptomatic relief and addressing the underlying source of respiratory distress, by adding them into their daily routine. Including these herbs in teas, infusions, or food preparations could provide a complementary and all-natural way to treat coughs.

CHAPTER FIVE

RECIPES AND FORMULATIONS USING HERBS

HERBAL INFUSIONS AND TEAS

For millennia, people from many different countries have prized herbal teas and infusions for their delicious flavors and medicinal qualities. Typically, plant parts like leaves, petals, seeds, or roots are infused into boiling water to create these mixtures. The resulting drinks have several health advantages in addition to being calming and fragrant. Herbal teas, as opposed to actual teas made from the Camellia sinensis plant, are devoid of caffeine and can be tailored to treat certain health issues or just improve general well-being.

SIMPLE RECIPES FOR HERBAL TEAS

Making simple yet satisfying herbal tea recipes is a fun way for people to learn more about the wide world of medicinal plants. Steeping dried herbs such as lavender, peppermint, or chamomile in hot water is a basic preparation. Renowned for its relaxing qualities, chamomile helps with digestion and encourages relaxation. Conversely, peppermint is renowned for both its cooling flavor and its digestive advantages. Calmness is enhanced by the invigorating scent of lavender. These fundamental recipes provide people with a starting point to experiment with various herbs and make custom mixes based on their tastes and medical requirements.

DRINKS TO PROMOTE RESPIRATORY HEALTH

Herbal infusions created especially to promote respiratory health are essential to overall wellness. The respiratory properties of ingredients like thyme, eucalyptus, and elderflower make them popular additions to these infusions. For example, thyme has long been used to treat respiratory problems and is known to have antibacterial qualities. Because of its well-known decongestant qualities, eucalyptus is a great option for respiratory support.

Because of its anti-inflammatory qualities, elderflower may also help relieve respiratory irritation. In addition to producing a tasty infusion, combining these herbs in an infusion has the medicinal potential to support respiratory health.

Herbal teas and infusions are an art form that offers a comprehensive approach to health and well-being, going beyond simple beverage selection. Simple herbal tea recipes provide a springboard for discovery, enabling people to enjoy the diverse range of tastes and health advantages that nature has to offer. Herbal infusions such as thyme, eucalyptus, and elderflower can be effective allies in preserving a healthy respiratory system when it comes to respiratory health. People who explore the world of herbal formulations not only find delicious flavors but also uncover the possibility of improving their general well-being and energy levels.

HERBAL TINCTURES AND SYRUPS

Herbal tinctures and syrups have long been valued for their therapeutic qualities since they provide a natural, all-encompassing approach to health and wellbeing. These concoctions use the medicinal properties of different plants, herbs, and other botanicals to treat particular medical issues. Syrups and tinctures are a well-liked category of herbal treatments, each with a distinct recipe and use.

HONEY-BASED COLD REMEDIES

Cough syrups with honey as an ingredient are a tried-and-true treatment for respiratory irritation and discomfort. The antibacterial and calming qualities of honey make it the ideal foundation for these syrups. These formulas contain carefully chosen herbs, including licorice root, elderberry, or thyme, to help not only reduce cough symptoms but also strengthen the immune system.

Because honey is thick, the medicinal ingredients stay in the throat longer, relieving coughing and discomfort over time.

ALCOHOL TINCTURES TO ALLEVIATE COUGH

One particularly useful way of delivering herbal remedies—especially for cough relief—is through alcohol tinctures. During the tincturing process, alcohol is used as a solvent to extract the active ingredients from herbs. This process guarantees a strong concentration of the beneficial qualities of herbs, facilitating the body's rapid and effective absorption. Echinacea, wild cherry bark, and elecampane are examples of herbs that are frequently used in alcohol tinctures to relieve coughs. In addition to being a potent extraction medium, the alcohol also functions as a preservative, extending the tincture's shelf life.

The skill of creating herbal syrups and alcohol tinctures is in the thoughtful selection and blending of herbs, taking into account each one's unique qualities and complementary effects. Herbalists and practitioners frequently construct well-balanced formulas that target certain health requirements by drawing on empirical facts as well as traditional knowledge. Maceration, infusion, or decoction are used in the process, depending on the desired result and the characteristics of the chosen herbs.

Moreover, herbal preparations have a holistic approach that goes beyond symptom relief. Numerous herbalists stress the significance of taking into account a person's total well-being and treating the underlying cause of health problems as opposed to just treating their symptoms. This philosophy, which strives for a holistic and long-term approach to health management, is strongly rooted in the manufacture of herbal tinctures and syrups.

Herbal tinctures and syrups offer successful remedies for a range of medical issues, representing a long history of complementary medicine. These recipes demonstrate the adaptability and effectiveness of herbal treatments, whether it's an alcohol tincture that targets respiratory problems or a honey-based cough syrup that provides calming relief.

CHAPTER SIX

USING HERBS IN EVERYDAY LIVING

USES OF MEDICINAL HERBS IN COOKING

Adding therapeutic herbs to regular cooking is a delicious and health-conscious method to add flavor to food while enjoying the many advantages of these amazing natural ingredients. Culinary herbs, like rosemary, basil, oregano, and thyme, give dishes essential nutrients and therapeutic qualities in addition to their unique aroma. For example, oregano has a high antioxidant content, and basil is well known for its anti-inflammatory qualities. Not only can these herbs improve food flavor, but they also enhance general health.

Trying out different herbal infusions in the kitchen is a great way to learn about different culinary cultures. Herbs like mint, cilantro, or sage can be added to oils or vinegar to give a distinctive and healthful edge to a variety of foods.

In addition, the use of medicinal herbs in recipes supports a holistic view of wellbeing, which recognizes that our diets affect our health in addition to satisfying our palates.

USING AROMATHERAPY TO IMPROVE RESPIRATORY HEALTH

Aromatherapy, a natural and comprehensive approach to respiratory health, is the therapeutic application of essential oils produced from medicinal herbs. Numerous herbs, including tea tree, peppermint, and eucalyptus, have strong fragrant components that are beneficial to the respiratory system. These essential oils can be inhaled using steam inhalations or diffusers to assist in clearing congestion, lessen inflammation, and support respiratory health in general.

Renowned for its decongestant qualities, eucalyptus can be especially useful in relieving respiratory pain. Breathing in its vapors facilitates airway opening and alleviates sinusitis and cold symptoms.

Because peppermint oil contains menthol, it has a cooling effect that helps relieve irritated respiratory tracts. A natural and non-invasive way to support respiratory health, including aromatherapy in everyday activities can be revitalizing and therapeutic.

STEAM INHALATIONS USING HERBS

Herbal steam inhalations are a well-established and efficacious technique for respiratory support that leverages the restorative qualities of medicinal herbs. Inhaling the herb-infused steam, which is frequently found in a bowl of hot water, helps to relieve congestion, calm irritated airways, and improve respiratory comfort. Herbs like lavender, chamomile, and eucalyptus are often used in steam inhalations.

Because of its antibacterial qualities, eucalyptus relieves respiratory distress in addition to helping to clear nasal passages. With its well-known relaxing properties, chamomile inhalation sessions can help lower tension and encourage relaxation. Apart from its soothing scent, lavender has anti-inflammatory qualities that can help with respiratory disorders.

Including herbal steam inhalations in a self-care regimen might be especially helpful in seasons when respiratory issues are common. Using the natural resources of the environment to support the respiratory system, this ancient method provides a calming and comprehensive approach to health.

CHAPTER SEVEN

GOOD LIVING PRACTICES
NUTRITION AND HYDRATION

Developing good nutrition and hydration practices is essential to keeping a healthy lifestyle. Our general health is strongly impacted by the food we eat, which has an impact on everything from immune system performance to energy levels. Adopting a diet that is well-balanced and rich in whole grains, lean meats, fruits, and vegetables gives the body the critical elements it needs to perform at its best. Because water is essential for digestion, vitamin absorption, and temperature regulation, staying properly hydrated is equally important.

Maintaining a healthy balance between nutrient-dense meals and adequate fluids supports long-lasting energy, helps with weight control, and enhances the body's general vitality.

EXERCISE FOR RESPIRATORY HEALTH

Including regular exercise in one's regimen is essential for sustaining respiratory health in addition to its cardiovascular health benefits. Aerobic exercise, like jogging, cycling, or brisk walking, increases lung capacity and efficiency. Furthermore, breathing exercises that target the respiratory system, like diaphragmatic breathing and deep inhalation techniques, can improve lung function and strengthen the respiratory muscles. Frequent exercise improves pulmonary resilience, which lowers the risk of respiratory diseases and lengthens life expectancy, in addition to improving general fitness.

TECHNIQUES FOR REDUCING STRESS

Considering the serious effects that long-term stress may have on one's physical and mental health, stress management is essential to leading a healthy lifestyle. Developing practical stress-reduction strategies is crucial for preserving equilibrium and advancing general health. By relaxing the neurological system, techniques including progressive muscle relaxation, deep breathing, and mindfulness meditation can help reduce stress. Taking part in enjoyable activities, such as hobbies or time spent in nature, can also help lower stress. A strong work-life balance and the development of social networks that support one another further increase resilience to life's setbacks, which eventually contributes to long-term well-being.

Adopting a healthy lifestyle calls for a comprehensive strategy that includes proper diet and hydration, exercise to support respiratory health and practical stress-reduction methods. These interrelated components support the general health of the body and mind, providing the groundwork for a happy and satisfying existence. Eating well-balanced meals regularly, drinking enough water, exercising to strengthen the lungs, and engaging in stress-reduction techniques all contribute to a balanced and long-lasting path to good health.

CHAPTER EIGHT

HOW TO AVOID COUGHS NATURALLY

DEVELOPING AN EFFECTIVE IMMUNE SYSTEM

Developing a robust immune system is essential for naturally avoiding coughs. The body's defense mechanism against different pathogens, such as bacteria and viruses that can cause respiratory infections and coughing, is the immune system. A strong immune system in balance can identify and repel these invaders with effectiveness. Sustaining immunological function primarily requires maintaining a healthy lifestyle. A healthy diet high in vitamins, minerals, and antioxidants, regular exercise, and enough sleep all support the immune system's general health. A healthy diet rich in immune-stimulating elements, such as zinc, vitamin D, and vitamin C, can help the body fight off infections and lessen the chance of coughing.

ENVIRONMENTAL ASPECTS TO TAKE INTO ACCOUNT

Natural cough prevention is greatly influenced by environmental factors. Respiratory health can be impacted by the settings we are exposed to and the air we breathe. It's critical to keep yourself safe from exposure to environmental pollutants like allergies, industrial pollutants, and cigarette smoke. These drugs have the potential to irritate the respiratory system, increasing a person's susceptibility to respiratory infections and coughing. A clean, well-ventilated living area is crucial for reducing indoor pollution exposure. Furthermore, maintaining a clean workplace and regularly washing your hands are two ways to practice good hygiene and stop the spread of infectious organisms that might cause coughing.

Apart from lifestyle and environmental factors, maintaining adequate hydration is a crucial component in the natural prevention of coughs. Maintaining proper hydration prevents the respiratory tract's mucous membranes from drying up and becoming more vulnerable to infections. Consuming enough fluids also aids in the body's normal functions, such as the removal of toxins and the movement of immune cells. Drinking water, herbal teas, and broths are great ways to stay properly hydrated and support the health of your respiratory system.

Moreover, natural cough prevention depends on stress management. Prolonged stress can have a deleterious effect on the immune system, increasing susceptibility to infections. Stress-reduction techniques including deep breathing exercises, meditation, and regular exercise can be incorporated to lessen the impacts of stress and promote a healthy immune system. A healthy, balanced way of living not only promotes general well-being but also helps ward against respiratory conditions like coughing.

Finally, a comprehensive strategy that takes into account both environmental influences and developing a robust immune system is needed to prevent coughs organically. Through the adoption of a health-conscious lifestyle, reducing pollution exposure, maintaining hydration, and effectively managing stress, people can strengthen their immunity to respiratory infections and lower their risk of coughing. These preventive actions benefit a person's general health in addition to their respiratory health.

www.ingramcontent.com/pod-product-compliance
Lightning Source LLC
Chambersburg PA
CBHW060848260726
48661CB00002B/679